Alzheimer's and Dementia

The Home-Care Family Guide for Elderly and Reconnecting Memories Using Activities

Jimmy D. Forest

D1528303

Contents

Alzheimer's and Dementia

Bluesource And Friends

This book is brought to you by Bluesource And Friends, a happy book publishing company.

Our motto is **"Happiness Within Pages"**

We promise to deliver amazing value to readers with our books.

We also appreciate honest book reviews from our readers.

Connect with us on our Facebook page www.facebook.com/bluesourceandfriends and stay tuned to our latest book promotions and free giveaways.

Don't forget to claim your FREE books!

Brain Teasers:

https://tinyurl.com/karenbrainteasers

Harry Potter Trivia:
https://tinyurl.com/wizardworldtrivia

Sherlock Puzzle Book (Volume 2)

https://tinyurl.com/Sherlockpuzzlebook2

Also check out our best seller book

https://tinyurl.com/lateralthinkingpuzzles

Introduction

Congratulations on getting *Alzheimer's and Dementia* and thank you for doing so.

If you have gotten this book, it's possible that you have a loved one who is suffering from dementia and you are in the role of the caregiver. It can be a daunting task having to care for someone who is suffering physically and losing mentally the characteristics that you may have known them for. Often dementia comes with mood swings, wandering issues, confusion and anxiety, and trouble communicating. Though there can be some medication that offers relief, unfortunately, symptoms tend to worsen as the disease progresses.

With this book, we hope to provide you with a series of important insights into dementia and what type of behavior your loved one may exhibit. With these behaviors are tips for you to stay in control and reduce stress if a situation should arise. The more prepared and positive you remain, the better your loved one may react which can mean a less volatile situation or emotional or violent outburst. By making your home a safe place and ensuring that all weak points are addressed, you can feel secure that your loved one is safe in their living quarters. With physical and mental activities, you can include in their schedule, as well as how to create a balanced and healthy diet, you can implement these tips to make it easier for you and your loved one to adjust with the effects of dementia.

There are plenty of books on this subject on the market, so thanks again for choosing this one!

Chapter 1: What Is Dementia & How Serious Is It?

Dementia does not refer to a specific disease. Rather, it's an overall broad term that refers to a group of symptoms that are associated with a general decline in cognitive and memory skills, that can impair a person's everyday activities. Most of the time, Alzheimer's disease accounts for almost 80% of the cases regarding dementia, but there can be other kinds as well depending on how serious your health condition is. For example, vascular dementia can occur after a stroke when a person is struggling with cognitive skills then. There are even some special conditions where dementia can be reversible, as such thyroid problems or severe vitamin deficiencies.

There are many health conditions that can cause dementia, but it's important to remember it as a symptom of the disease. It's mistakenly sometimes referred to as a natural part of the aging process, but it's important to know that severe gaps in memory and loss of cognitive skills is not normal, but is most likely associated with a neurodegenerative condition. Symptoms of dementia can vary greatly and do not have to be alike for any two people. But most of the following functions tend to be impaired:

- reasoning and judgment skills
- visual perception
- verbal communication
- memory and recall
- ability to focus on a task
- clear thinking

Most types of dementia tend to be progressive, which means the symptoms start out very slowly but then tend to become worse over time. That can be a sign of the condition progressing. There is still research being done on how dementia may run in families. Certain types of dementia are inherited as a single gene, though every human tends to have a combination of genes that increases or decreases their risk of developing dementia in much less direct ways. Alzheimer's studies reveal that many family members can be affected by the disease over successive generations. There could be a mutation that is passed from parent to child.

Chapter 2: Seeking Treatment

There is no one test to determine if someone has dementia, which is why it's so important to be looking for clues into someone's condition. Even if someone is experiencing short term dementia, such as constantly forgetting appointments or where they put items, or how to do certain tasks, that's still a clue of what could be the onset of dementia. Sometimes, other people do have memory recall issues and it doesn't have to be dementia or linked with any other disease. But if you notice memory difficulties or a sudden decline in cognitive skills, the most important thing is to visit a doctor to determine the cause.

A professional evaluation from a licensed health care provider could provide you answers regarding dementia and how far it has progressed. Often cases of Alzheimer's are diagnosed based on a physical examination, lab tests, tests of mental skills, a careful medical history check, and observing the day to day functioning behavior and cognitive recall. It can still be hard for doctors to determine the exact type of dementia, because there are often symptoms that overlap. You may have to see a neurologist or geriatrician for further testing to develop a path of treatment. A scan of your brain could show how far the disease has progressed.

Even an early diagnosis of dementia could help the person get available treatment or be enrolled in clinical trials or studies to try and reverse the memory loss. The earlier you notice it, the better you can fight against it with exercise and cognitive activities. Of course, a diagnosis is important to plan for the future. If you have a loved one living alone, you may want to make changes to their living situation to assure they are not alone. If they are already living with you, it still requires certain adjustments and ensuring their safety in the home.

Alzheimer's and Dementia

Treatment of dementia depends on its cause. If it's progressive dementia such as Alzheimer's, there sadly is no cure or treatment that stops its progression. Unfortunately, the symptoms of dementia seem to only get worse with time when it comes to Alzheimer's patients. But there can be drugs that help to improve symptoms. Even non-drug therapies are encouraged to keep patients in a routine and encourage new activities. It could help with their memory and recall skills and encourage them to use their cognitive skills despite the mental decline.

It could be that the cure for dementia is found for future generations, which is why research funding and participation in clinical trials is so important. If your loved one consents to be involved in medical trials, that is a great way to ensure that their experience battling dementia can be used for science to help future patients.

Chapter 3: Common Dementia Behavior

Dementia is a very individualized journey with no two progressions of the disease quite alike. At the onset of dementia, it often seems harmless with just the person forgetting little details or words, or losing things. They still seem like themselves and it can seem like "normal" aging symptoms. But eventually, as dementia worsens, a number of behaviors present itself and makes it harder for the person to live their life and perform everyday tasks.

Some of these behaviors include but are not limited to:

Confusion: This is usually one of the first signs of dementia and begins with your loved one forgetting words, common information, or having trouble remembering new information. The initial forgetfulness may seem harmless but as dementia progresses, the confusion becomes worse and your

14

loved one may forget who the people in their life are, where they are, and what year it is. They may forget things about their past and experiences and memories that were dear to them. This confusion can be hard to combat, so try and be as reassuring as you can as you gently talk to your loved one and validate their feelings regarding their emotions. Sometimes repeating to them the facts is unhelpful—they simply cannot remember.

Changes in eating habits: Often, people with dementia may lose weight because they forget to eat or suddenly change their eating habits. They may not like foods they once loved, or can be feeling too morose or anxious to eat a full meal like they once did. When this happens, you want to be sure you're providing your loved one with meals and beverages that are healthy and filling, and keeping a close eye on them to ensure they're being eaten. If they lose too much weight, be sure you consult their doctor on supplements or medication changes.

Lack of hygiene: People with middle-stage dementia stop caring about their appearance as well. Often, if they are housebound, they may not bother to brush their hair, change their clothes, or bother to take a shower or bath for many days. When you notice the decline in these habits, you want to be sure you are stepping in and gently encouraging them to continue. Make it a routine that you and your loved one do together so that they feel accomplished. If it seems like they've forgotten how to, work with them to demonstrate and mimic the actions to help them remember.

Sundowning: This is a term that is used regarding the agitated or anxious behavior that dementia patients exhibit in the early evening. Research believes it's because they tend to be exhausted mentally by all the activities throughout the day. Combine that with the mental confusion, they may be unable to voice their concerns or properly express their mental and physical exhaustion. In order to try and avoid this stressful "witching hour," try and avoid strenuous

16

activities like bathing, exercise, or mealtimes at this time. Instead, make it a quiet time where the person can relax, read, or spend some time alone as they get ready for bed. Avoid sugar and caffeine around this time because it could only exacerbate their behavior. Remain calm if mood changes occur, and remind yourself that your loved one needs validation about their feelings.

Accusations and Bitterness: Even the most good-natured individuals can experience phases of accusations and bitterly lashing out when they are going through dementia. Often, they will lash out at caregivers or family members and accuse them of lying or withholding information from them. Maybe they'll accuse them of taking their things or keeping them cooped up and not letting them live freely like they once were. Remember when these phases occur, it's not a personal attack towards you—it's dementia, not your loved one. Don't try to argue, but try and shift the conversation and distract them with another topic or task. Re-direction is going to be a key tool

17

when dealing with dementia patients, because it may help to prevent escalations in arguments.

Hand-Wringing, Pacing, Rocking Back and Forth: These physical motions can be a way that a dementia patient manifests their anxiety. They could become restless and be triggered by any new factors in their environment or new emotions and feelings. If you notice these signs, take the time to talk to your loved one and see what is causing their anxiety. Try to divert their attention to calm them down, and recommend a calming activity like a walk or listening to music.

Repeating False Stories: Your loved one could be repeating stories that never happened but ones that they seem to firmly believe did. These are manifested in hallucinations or delusions based on false beliefs. It could be overall confusion regarding the passage of time or filling in the gaps of their memory, as they've lost the original ones about what has happened to them in their life. When this occurs, try to gently tell your loved one that this isn't true, and have them look through old photographs or a scrapbook of memories and see what they may remember. But more often than not, it's not worth the energy to argue with the dementia patient, because it may aggravate them even more. This could lead to an argument or frustration that is more difficult for you to manage. If it gives them comfort to relay these false stories, then let them continue to do so.

Wandering and Leaving the House Unassisted:
Unfortunately, wandering is a very common type of behavior in dementia patients, even if it seems harmless and your loved one is saying they are doing it for innocent reasons like using the bathroom or looking for their medication. It's important that when wandering occurs, someone is there monitoring your loved one full-time. We'll discuss more on this in a later chapter and mention safety tips you should be aware of and implement.

Chapter 4: Fear of Violence

It can be overwhelming to know how to respond when your loved one with dementia is behaving aggressively. Sometimes their behavior can be physically or mentally exhausting, and it can be very distressing for caregivers. This type of behavior may be linked to the individual's personality before they developed dementia, but aggression can show up in individuals regardless of their previous personality type. It can include verbal or physical behavior, and a mix of screaming, shouting, making threats, hitting, biting, or pushing and shoving.

Often this physical aggression can be manifested due to the patient's frustration. They may be unable to recognize their needs, or know how to fulfill them or communicate well enough to share what they desire with you as the caregiver. There can be many causes of this violent behavior, such as:

- **Side effects of medication and dosage changes:** This can lead the person to feel confused and drowsy and maybe push back their already poor communication skills

- **Overwhelming environment:** Maybe they feel the area they are living in is not compatible with their likes. It could be too noisy or bright, or busy and loud. Or maybe it's too quiet and boring and the quiet is what makes them anxious.

- **Failing hearing or vision:** Loss of functioning senses can make any person feel overwhelmed and lost, even more so someone with dementia who is struggling to rely on their mental abilities.

- **Hallucinations:** These delusions can be frightening for your loved one, and lead them to feel quite sure that what they saw is real. If you or another family member dares to question the validity of them, your loved one

may become more aggressive at being
questioned.

- **In pain or discomfort:** Maybe your loved
  one is having some physical discomfort that
  they cannot explain. Be sure they are going for
  regular check-ups and having routine physical
  examinations to ensure no physical
  discomfort is missed.

- **Loss of agency:** Losing the ability to care for
  yourself and make your own decisions can be
  frustrating, and your loved one may feel
  depressed or disgruntled about how much
  they cannot do.

When sessions of aggressiveness occur, it's important
you know how to cope for your own sake and the
sake of your loved one. Before reacting, take a deep
breath and give the person some space. Staying calm
is key, because you don't want to show your
frustration or anger—that could possibly make the
situation worse and escalate the emotions. Try to

reserve showing any fear or anxiety because this could cause the person's agitation to worsen. If you feel threatened though, you should leave the situation and call for some help. Ensure that you are safe because your safety is very important.

Give the person plenty of space and time. Do not try to initiate physical contact, because the person may find it threatening. A good tip is to keep your body posture and body language similar to the other person's. If they're sitting down, you should too. Mimic their body language so it puts them at ease and does not make you seem like a threat. Maintaining eye contact is another good idea.

Try and reassure the person and acknowledge their feelings. If they are angry, mention why they feel that way. If they feel scared, reassure them that they are safe and that this is their home. Remind yourself that the person is not meaning to lash out at you personally, but they must have some reason to communicate with you even if that is coming out in a violent outburst. Try and distract the person with another topic or a task that may relax them.

When the violent behavior has passed, remind yourself not to punish the person for their behavior or hold it against them. In most cases, their judgment has eroded, so they don't even realize what they have done or understand why it was dangerous. Try to be as reassuring as you can, and maintain the same routine and demeanor towards them. Focus on the person and how they are feeling and if they have adjusted to normal.

In your case as the caregiver, it could be beneficial for you to talk to someone about how you're feeling, whether that's other family members, a counselor or support worker, or the general physician. If you don't talk about your feelings, it may be harder for you to focus and push aside negative feelings to care for your loved one. Be sure you're taking time for yourself to relax and experience self-care. That means some time off from your duties and spending time with your own friends and family to put you at ease.

Your physician or counselor could help you identify steps for managing aggressive behavior in your loved one. This could help you notice signs of trouble. Identifying the problem is important therefore, take the time to think over what could be bringing out this reaction in your dementia patient. Is it something about their living situation? Are they in pain or having some discomfort? Is it because of their social environment, or is it because they are not getting enough socialization? When and where did this situation begin? Were there other people involved? Look for any patterns that you noticed in the behavior. Sometimes keeping a diary or jotting down anything about when the aggressive behavior begins could help you notice patterns. Identify how the person reacts, and try to develop a strategy. If you need to, get your patient's physician or counselor involved if you feel the situation has not gotten better.

Chapter 5: Working With Memory

There is a general consensus among health advisors that mental stimulation could slow the decline of dementia and help with memory recall. Many studies have found that participants who received routine cognitive stimulation were able to interact and communicate better than they previously were, and it improved their overall quality of life. Now, it all depends on what stage of dementia your loved one is at. If they are in mild or moderate stages, short-term improvements may be possible to prevent further cognitive decline. If dementia has further progressed, don't feel guilty if the activities are not helping them or you're not seeing progress.

The great thing about cognitive stimulation is that it can be done either in a group setting or individually. If your loved one is in a nursing home or residential care facility, then the staff has probably set up activities to keep residents mentally engaged. But if your loved one lives with you as their caregiver, you can address their individual needs and find activities based on their interests and level of skill. This one-on-one connection is very valuable as you take the time to work with your loved one.

There are a variety of activities you can do to keep your loved one mentally stimulated.

- **Creative Activities:** painting, arts and crafts projects, knitting, embroidery, playing music or singing.

  - These activities are a great way to reinforce your loved one's creative skills, such as if they loved to play an instrument or knit. It can be hard for them to recall these skills so be patient and work alongside them, encouraging them if they have forgotten some steps. Taking a class at your local community center with them is a great way to have a social outing and still encourage their creative side.

Thinking Activities: reading, puzzles, board games, crossword puzzles, Scrabble, maze puzzles.

- These types of activities are great to encourage cognitive activity and "exercise" the brain. They can be solitary activities that you give your loved one while you work on something else, or something that you can work on together. Help them when necessary if they get stumped, but always be encouraging to them if they feel frustrated they cannot do it themselves.

Physical Activities: taking a walk, dancing, exercising, yoga, stretching.

- Engaging in physical activity is a great way to encourage exercise and monitor your loved one's flexibility and endurance. Of course, these types of activities may be hindered with age and physical conditions, but even just a calming walk around the block or going to a yoga class for seniors could help your loved one stay mentally alert. Exercise has tons of benefits including boosting your energy level, providing a better night's sleep, and improving your mood. Of course, you don't want to leave your loved one alone walking around if they have severe dementia or wandering issues. Be sure to accompany them, or that they are always under supervision if they are taking a class. Be sure the instructor or front desk associate knows that your loved one should always remain inside, and to call you if they become agitated or are trying to wander off.

Social Activities: senior center activities, community center classes, visiting with friends or family.

Alzheimer's and Dementia

- Depending on how progressive your loved one's dementia is, how comfortable they feel in social settings can vary. If it's still mild, they may feel fine in social settings and conversing with other people for longer lengths of time. If dementia has progressed, they may suddenly forget who the people in the group are, or feel unsafe and become agitated. It's up to you as a caregiver to realize their level and ensure they never feel scared or uncomfortable in a group setting. If you need to, you can accompany them to classes occurring at your local community center or senior center, so that you are nearby in case they become frustrated or forget where they are. Visiting with family and friends can also put people at ease, but be sure the visits are monitored and are not too lengthy. You don't want to make your loved one feel that they have to entertain for long lengths of time, or have a topic come up that makes them angry or upset.

Chores: setting the table, putting out pet food, folding the laundry, cleaning up, doing the dishes.

- Even if your loved one lives with you and isn't responsible for household chores, keeping them involved is a great way to make them feel capable. It could be something as simple as setting the table for dinner or helping you wash dishes afterward. Continuing this routine can make them feel involved and responsible, and reduce their feelings of helplessness. Always be there to assist.

Daily Living Activities: brushing teeth, eating, getting dressed, taking a shower or bath.

- It's a great idea to constantly be going over these with your loved one to ensure they are able to properly perform them. Sometimes they may walk out of the bathroom without brushing their teeth, or become overwhelmed when taking a shower. Make sure you're there to guide them and encourage them, but never make them feel like they are failing by forgetting certain steps.

Reminiscence Therapy: looking at photo albums, telling stories from the past, re-reading old letters, creating a scrapbook, continuing a family tradition of certain activities or meals.

- These types of activities can be great to help your loved one with memory recall. They don't have to remember specific details, but it's a great way to take a trip down memory lane and see what they remember without pressuring them. Studies have shown that these types of activities can greatly improve memory recall in individuals with dementia.

Alzheimer's and Dementia

But you want to be sure it's done naturally and made to feel like a relaxing activity, instead of an activity that's being graded.

Chapter 6: Speech and Communication Issues

Unless you are educated or studied speech and communicative behavior, it can be very hard to communicate with someone who has dementia. After communicating with healthy people who are able to strongly communicate their thoughts, it can be very difficult to be patient and change your style when speaking to your loved one who has dementia. But the more patient you are, the better your relationship with your loved one will be, and hopefully add less stress to your life as you care for the person.

Here are some tips to help you set up a positive and successful interaction as you communicate with the person with dementia.

Ensure there are no distractions. People with dementia can be distracted by even the littlest things like if the television is on, or if there's noise coming from the corner of the room. If you want to speak to the person and ensure you are being listened, limit any distractions and potential noise. Move to a quieter room if you need to. Get the person's attention by addressing their name and gently reminding them who you are. If they're sitting down, you should as well to get to their eye level and maintain eye contact.

Show a positive mood. Remember, body language is key when speaking to someone, and you never know cues your loved one is picking up, even with dementia. That's why it's so important to set a positive mood for your loved one, and keep a pleasant tone and relaxed body language. The tone of your voice and your facial expressions can convey a lot to someone, so you want to always be gentle and convey respect and affection. Being unnecessarily harsh or loud may only make the person cower and fear you.

Alzheimer's and Dementia

Be clear and concise. You want to speak slowly and in a reassuring tone, and use simple words and sentence structures. The clearer and more concise you are, it will be much easier for the person to grasp your directions. If they don't show they've understood the first time, repeat your words or your question, but be sure you don't give away impatience or frustration in your tone. If the person still does not understand, re-phrase your question in a different way.

Ask simple questions with a "yes" or "no" answer. You want to keep your questions to one at a time, and enure they have simple yes or no answers to avoid confusion. Open-ended questions may only frustrate the person if they are unable to form a response or recall the answer. It's better to say the options that you're giving so the person can make a clear choice. For example, you can ask, "Do you want to have a salad for lunch or a grilled cheese sandwich?" This gives the two options clearly, and the person hears them so they can repeat which they prefer. If you say something open-ended like, "What would you like for lunch?" the number of unlimited options could confuse them.

Gently help them through activities by using a sequence of steps. This can help your loved one find tasks more manageable, even the simple things like getting dressed in the morning. Gently remind them of the series of steps such as, "Pick out which shirt you want to wear today," and then, "Don't forget to wear socks with your shoes." These gentle clues will help them in the process and avoid making them feel ashamed if they forgot any steps.

If the person becomes frustrated, distract them and re-direct their attention. Depending on your loved one's mood or level of discomfort with what you are talking about or doing, they could become agitated or upset. That's when it's key you change the subject, or get them into a different environment to distract them. Suggest going for a walk or getting something to eat from the kitchen. Be sure you tell them you understand how they feel. For example, you can say something like, "I didn't mean to bring up something that makes you angry. Let's go for a walk instead." If you acknowledge their feelings, it could help them move past it and follow your directions to a new task.

Be affectionate. People with dementia often feel unsure of themselves and the situation around them. They may confuse reality with things that never happened and feel convinced that those events did occur. The best way that you can approach someone with dementia is with affection. Stay focused on their feelings and respond verbally with comfort and reassurance. Sometimes physical affection can help calm them down, whether it's holding hands or a hug, to remind them of your relationship and how much you care about them. A sense of humor can help, but be sure you're not laughing at the person's expense or making a joke about them.

Alzheimer's and Dementia

Chapter 7: Home Hazards

Your loved one with dementia can live peacefully in your home as long as you are aware of hazards and have taken the appropriate safety measures. Due to impaired judgment and confused behavior, it's important that dementia patients are protected from certain hazards in the home. You never want to leave an opportunity for an accident to occur, which can be serious neglect on your part if you have not addressed weak spots in your home.

Here are some home safety tips to ensure you have made your living area safe for your loved one with Alzheimer's or dementia.

Carefully evaluate each room in your home and the outdoors. A person with dementia may wander throughout the home and explore areas they are not supposed to, even if you have set limits for them. It's important you pay attention to all areas including

41

basements, garages, or outside areas and determine if anything needs special accommodations. Also be aware of areas where you keep medicines, cleaning supplies, any chemicals or tools, which will need to be blocked off.

Pay careful attention to the safety hazards in the kitchen. Whether it's knives, the stove, or the microwave, take time to catalog the safety hazards in the kitchen. You may have to take specific steps to handle each hazard differently. For example, be sure you have a safety lock on the drawers to make sure your knife drawer or medicine cabinet is locked. Install a gas shut-off valve or a breaker near the stove and be sure it's turned off after use, so the individual with dementia cannot turn on the stove. You can even child-lock the knobs. Be sure there aren't cooking seasonings like salt or sugar out on the table in glass jars which could get broken. This often tends to be the most dangerous area of the house, so you want to give it a thorough assessment.

Be sure all your safety devices are working properly. You want to be sure you have smoke and carbon monoxide detectors installed in the home in working order. Have a fire extinguisher handy if you have space. We often don't think about these devices, but just their presence saves lives! And that can only happen if they are working, so be sure to check the batteries!

Install extra lights and make sure all areas of access are well-lit. As we mentioned, dementia patients can often wander, so it's important these areas of your home are well-lit. That includes doorways, entryways, stairways, and even areas between rooms. Install extra lights or brighter lights in areas where they need them to avoid any potential falls. Be sure to remove tripping hazards to prevent any accidents. You want every path that your loved one may take to the restroom, or to any other area of the house, to be free of barriers and brightly lit.

Injury-proof the bathroom. This can be an area of accidental slips and falls if it's not secure for your loved one's use. Have a walk-in shower instead of a high edge bathtub to make it easier for your dementia patient to get in and out, and install grab bars so they can safely do so. Be very aware of slippery floor tiles, and add textured stickers or water-proof stickers instead of rugs that could slip.

Remove and disable any guns and weapons from your home. If you have a firearm in your home, it's essential that you keep it locked and hidden away at all times. Having such a thing in the home of a person with dementia can lead to all sorts of tragic situations if they come across it. They could mistakenly see another family member as an intruder, or even turn it on themselves. It's very, very important that firearms are always disabled or removed entirely from the vicinity.

Be sure all chemicals are locked away safely.
Cleaning supplies, cleaning ammonia, laundry
detergent "pads," and bleach can all be dangerous if a
dementia patient stumbles upon them. Ensure all
those items are kept in hard to reach places or in
locked shelves where your loved one cannot get a
hold of them. There also could be dangerous
substances in your garage such as spray paint or paint
thinner. You want to be sure those are kept out of
reach as well.

**Watch for extreme temperatures of water and
food.** A person with dementia may forget to wait
until their bath cools down, or their food is cool
enough to eat. You can install a thermometer in your
bathtub or get auto-adjusted shower controls to
ensure they aren't going to hurt themselves with
scalding water.

Have a list of emergency contacts. Be sure there is
a visible list of emergency phone numbers and

addresses for loved ones, doctors, local police and fire department, hospitals, and a poison control center. Ensure everyone in the house knows where this list is as well as any other caretakers who may be watching your loved one in your absence. No matter how much you're preparing to prevent emergencies, it's always best to know who to call if there is one.

Chapter 8: Food and Nutrition for Dementia

Mealtimes can be a battle with a loved one who has dementia. As a person's dementia progresses, they may forget to eat, have difficulty with utensils, or throw fits regarding food choices and what they're being served. Despite these hurdles, any doctor will tell you that proper nutrition is important to keep your loved one healthy and strong. Poor nutrition can offer other health hurdles such as diabetes, behavioral issues, or cause weight loss. Not only that, it's important for you to stay healthy as a caregiver too! You are taking on the extra responsibility of caring for a loved one, which means you need your energy and to take care of yourself too.

You want to have a balanced diet with a variety of foods. That includes things like fresh fruits and vegetables, whole grains, lean, high-protein meats, and low-fat dairy products. Always be sure to follow the diet that your dementia patient's physician or nutritionist advises. More than likely, they will recommend you limit foods with high cholesterol and high saturated fat content. High saturated fat can increase your risk of cardiovascular disease. Avoid refined sugars as well, because they can be very harmful to patients at risk for diabetes. Instead, focus on healthy sweet options like fresh, ripe fruit, honey, or agave nectar as a topping on yogurt or oatmeal. If your loved one has high blood pressure issues, you also want to avoid using too much salt, which can cause hypertension. Instead, use natural spices as an alternative when seasoning your food.

It's also important that your loved one stays hydrated and has plenty of water. Often with the memory loss and symptoms of dementia, patients tend to forget to drink enough water and can be negligent about staying hydrated. But dehydration can lead to many other issues such as rapid heartbeat and breathing, faintness and lethargy, feeling dizzy, and having urinary problems. Be sure you are offering your loved one enough water throughout the day, filling up their water bottle, and monitoring their intake. You also want to give foods with high liquid content such as soups, milkshakes, healthy smoothies, and fresh fruit.

Often as dementia progresses, patients tend to lose their appetite, and weight loss can be an area of concern. In this case, the doctor may suggest supplementing in between meals with protein drinks or bars that could provide extra calories. Keep in mind the opposite can occur too where the person may not remember they ate! In that case, don't keep reminding them that they already ate if they clearly cannot remember. Instead, offer several short meals over time, such as cereal, followed by a slice of toast, and then a bowl of fresh fruit. Have healthy snacks handy if they say they are hungry even if they just ate. That way, at least they're eating something healthy!

It's also important you recognize any possible causes of poor appetite that may occur in your dementia patient. This can occur when your loved one doesn't recognize a new food or is unwilling to test it. Eating could also be painful if there are dental or denture issues, so be sure you are visiting the dentist regularly. As dementia worsens, patients sense of smell and taste often worsen, so they may feel like their food has become bland and lose their appetite. New medications or changes in dosage can also affect appetite. When you notice significant decreases in appetite, it's important you contact the patient's doctor to discuss what to do.

With all these difficulties that can occur, mealtime can be trying. In order to make meals easier, here are some tips you can try to implement.

Avoid distractions. As we've mentioned before, one of the symptoms of dementia can be difficulty focusing on a task. That's why you want to aim to make mealtimes as peaceful as possible without outside distractions or the television on. Be sure your area is quiet, and avoid having distractions around like paperwork or other tasks that could distract your loved one from their meal.

Be sure you've checked the food temperature before serving. Dementia patients often have difficulty gauging the temperature of something. This could mean burning themselves if they touch a hot plate, or drink scalding soup or coffee. As the caregiver, be sure you're testing the temperature of the foods and beverages before serving. If you serve it hot, even if you tell them to wait a few minutes until it cools, they may not, which could lead to a burn or injury.

Encourage independence when eating. Keep in mind what the person's abilities are. If they can eat with a spoon and fork, then encourage them to eat what they can by themselves. If they cannot use utensils, serve finger-friendly foods, so they can feel independent by still feeding themselves. Don't worry so much about neatness, but let them eat as much as they can by themselves. Be sure the food you prepare isn't hard to swallow or a choking hazard.

Use a place setting where the food is easily distinguished from the plate. Often changes in visual and spatial abilities can make it hard for a dementia patient to distinguish their food on the plate. Avoid patterned dishes that make it hard to see the food clearly. It can help to use plain white dishes and bowls so your loved one can clearly see the food color, texture, and portion size.

Be open to changes in food preferences.
Remember that dementia can cause the individual to suddenly change their mind regarding certain foods. This means your loved one might suddenly develop a taste for food they never liked before, or reject foods

that they have loved forever. Remember, stay in a positive attitude and be flexible to these changes!

Eat together as a family if you can. Try and make mealtimes as enjoyable and as relaxing as you can, to put all family members at ease with one another. This way, everyone looks forward to the experience of spending time together and sharing a delicious and healthy meal. This will make it a time that your loved one actually looks forward to instead of dreading.

Give the person enough time to eat. The last thing you want to do is rush the person eating and make mealtime an even more stressful situation. Instead, be aware that your dementia patient may take longer to eat. Their attention may wander, they may get lost in their thoughts, so it may take them extra time to taste and carefully chew each bite of food. It could sometimes take an hour or longer for them to finish a meal and feel satisfied they ate. Be patient and be sure you've scheduled enough time for their meal.

Alzheimer's and Dementia

Chapter 9: Daily Exercises

Just like with nutrition and dietary requirements, you want to be sure you've spoken to your loved one's doctor regarding physical exercise. There may be some health concerns regarding individual physical conditions, but most doctors will recommend non-strenuous exercise, which can improve flexibility, blood circulation, strength, and quality of sleep. It's a great mood booster and energy booster too! The more limber and active your loved one is in their senior years, the more they can remain agile for longer and have an active and improved quality of life.

It may be tough at first to encourage your loved one to participate in exercise, especially if they previously avoided it. To combat this, treat it like a fun activity instead of a chore, such as a dance party or a yoga session with relaxing music. It might help if you exercise with them as well. This can give them more confidence in case they forget the steps, and they can mimic your movements. Plus, isn't it always more fun to exercise with a friend?

It doesn't have to be a complex workout or even require physically leaving your house. It's simply about making the time and putting in some effort. For beginners, starting with just 10 to 15 minutes a few times a week is ideal, and then maybe scheduling it for 20 to 25-minute block sessions every other day. You don't want to push too hard initially, because that could risk injury.

There are many benefits of exercise as we mentioned above, and you may soon see improvements in your loved one's overall health. These include things like:

- slowing mental decline
- reducing the risk of depression
- improving heart health
- helping them sleep faster and improving the quality of sleep

- reducing constipation and digestive issues
- improving balance and flexibility
- reducing stress and improving mood
- reducing episodes of wandering or agitation due to mood changes

Safety is first and foremost, which is why you want to be sure to speak to the doctor before making any changes in your loved one's physical routine. Be sure you are present and monitoring the level of exertion, so it is a comfortable pace. Ensure they are well hydrated and taking breaks as necessary. If you notice signs of weakness, dizziness, or any pain, stop immediately and rest.

What kind of simple to moderate exercises can be performed by seniors with dementia? Here are some suggestions that you can try.

- **Walking:** This is a simple exercise that we often don't even think of as exercise! But just a walk around the house, in the yard, or down the block can be a great way to get fresh air, stretch your limbs, and expend some energy. If your loved one is reluctant to exercising, disguise it in a way that can get them involved, such as taking the dog for a walk or walking down the street to a friend's house.

- **Working on balance:** Stay balanced in a standing position by holding what you need for support, and then try to stay balanced against the wall in a sitting position. This activity can improve balance and posture over time.

- **Stretching:** Simply stretching your body can help to relax stiff muscles and ease the pain in your joints. It can be done with assistance or done independently. Sometimes going for a massage can be a great way to ease sore limbs too!

- **Yoga, Pilates, or Tai Chi:** These exercises tend to be less cardio and more stretching, which can be ideal for senior citizens. Try following a routine online or joining a local class in your gym. They can be adapted as necessary based on your loved one's physical needs.

- **Household chores:** These can be a great way to "sneak" in exercise for your loved one without them knowing. It allows them to feel involved in the housework and capable of doing their share. Things like dusting around the house, light vacuuming, and washing dishes all require motor activity.

- **Gardening:** If your loved one has a green thumb and loves to garden, this is a great activity for them to be involved in. It's exercise without feeling like a chore! Pulling weeds, shoveling, or raking can be a great workout, and you can watch your vegetable garden and flowers grow too!

- **Water exercises:** These are considered great for senior citizens, because there is no stress on the joints when underwater. It's a great way to reduce the symptoms of arthritis and the pressure on your joints. Water also acts as a form of resistance, so you can perform strength exercises without weights! Your local gym or senior center should offer an array of water aerobic classes for senior citizens.

- **Dancing:** This can be a great social activity that also incorporates physical exercise. If your loved one enjoys dancing or a certain style like the salsa or waltz, this is a great way to get them on their feet again! You can play the music at home and have your own dance party, or see if your local senior center or

retirement center has dancing classes or
parties that your loved one can attend.

Chapter 10: Wandering Issues

People with dementia often tend to walk aimlessly. The reasons could be the side effect of certain medications, boredom in their environment, they claim to be "looking for something" or someone despite being confused about where that person or thing is. They may claim they are hungry, thirsty, or need to use the restroom. This type of behavior can be very unsettling for caregivers and frightening, especially if you're in a home with stairs or hazards around the corner. It's important to take the time to try and discover any triggers regarding wandering, and take the appropriate steps to minimize any potential risk.

Here are some tips that may help you if you have a loved one who tends to wander.

- Add some child-safe plastic covers to doorknobs or drawers you do not want the person getting into, such as medicine drawers, and cutlery or knife drawers.

- Be sure the person is getting regular exercise. This could make them feel less restless, that they've had time to explore the indoors or outdoors that day, and like they do not need to go wandering for curiosity's sake.

- Install home security or monitoring system that can watch over the person, especially if you are away from home or no one is at home to watch them. If the system has a speaker system so you can talk to the person and give them directions, it is a great addition to calm them if they seem to be wandering around the house.

- Look into a GPS devise that can be used to track the person's whereabouts if they wander off. They can be added to their watch or worn as a necklace to ensure you can find them if they do wander off.

- Use barriers like a curtain or a visible STOP sign to remind your loved one that they should not go past this point.

- Be sure your loved one is wearing an ID bracelet. That way, if they wander off and cannot recall their name or give identifying information, their name and address can be identified by people. Have a recent photo of your loved one for identification purposes.

- Inform your neighbors about the wandering issues and be sure they know to contact you if they spot the person in the yard or leaving the vicinity of the home.

- Try installing new locks that require a different key. Try to position them high or low on the door, because people with dementia often simply look at their eye level. Be sure to give keys to all other family members to account for potential fire or safety concerns. You don't want to make it difficult for other household members!

Chapter 11: Handling Mood Changes

With caring for dementia patients, you have to be watchful of mood changes that can occur. Whether that's due to medication side effects, frustration at their declining cognitive skills, or simply a bad mood that day, these mood swings can appear suddenly. They could include moods like:

- apathy
- depression
- frustration
- anger
- agitation
- nervousness
- anxiety or fear
- overreaction
- hysteria
- sadness

These mood changes can make it hard for you to gauge how to handle your loved one. It's important that you know what to do and do not appear surprised or disappointed at their mood swings. That could escalate their behavior even more. Remind yourself that it's not the person's fault—the dementia is overcoming their senses and often making their emotions volatile.

Here are some tips we can offer you on how to cope with mood swings for a smoother situation, for you and your loved one with dementia.

Take complaints of pain seriously. If the person is saying they are hurt or having pain, don't be quick to ignore it even if they do have a tendency to say untrue things or makeup stories. You never want the case to be that they are hurt and it was overlooked. Take the time to ask them how they feel—are they tired? Hungry? Sleepy? Thirsty? Where does it hurt? Check to see how they are feeling and ensure there aren't any physical marks or bruises on their body.

Make sure the person has enough activities. Sometimes mood swings can occur because of boredom or tiredness. Ensure that your loved one has enough activities to do throughout the day, with enough time to rest and nap too. Are they getting enough exercise? Do they prefer a morning or evening walk? Do they like to be indoors or outdoors? Do they have enough engaging mental activities like reading or doing puzzles to keep them entertained? Make sure their routine has enough activities to keep them entertained, as well as time to relax and unwind. You want to have a schedule they are comfortable with and not make any sudden changes which could cause frustration.

Work with them through the tasks that frustrate them. Often if a person is unable to remember how to do something, they may lash out and have a mood swing. When you feel something like this coming on or recognize they are feeling insecure about a certain task, like helping set the table or combing their hair, take the time to complete the task with them. This will refresh their memory and build their confidence.

Create a calm and peaceful environment. Even if you have a busy home life with many people coming in and out, ensure that the person with dementia always feels the home is a safe and inviting place. This might mean setting something like "quiet hours" to ensure they are not disturbed, or directing children or teenagers to play in another part of the house if the noise level bothers your loved one. Sudden noise or interruptions in their routine could cause mood changes in your loved one, so be sure you are setting routines that put them at ease as not to startle them.

Offer a distraction. This might seem like an avoidance tactic, but sometimes just changing the subject and offering a distraction may help you avoid

69

a major meltdown and emotional situation. See if they want a snack or a drink, or want to take a walk around the house or outside. Maybe you can mention you have an errand to run or a task to complete and they can assist. Sometimes just getting their mind off the topic could ease them back into their good mood.

Keep your goodbyes short. Often if you are leaving the house for an errand or have to say goodbye to your loved one with dementia for a few hours, this goodbye can cause a great deal of anxiety in them. You may hear from the person who is watching them that they instantly have a mood change and are difficult to deal with for a while afterward. In order to avoid this change in behavior, make your goodbyes short to avoid upsetting them. Don't tell the person you are going to be leaving repeatedly, because that may stress them out even more. Act natural and then mention that you will be going and will see them in a few hours. This makes it easier for them as they are not dwelling over your departure.

When in doubt, get help. If you feel your loved one is having difficulty with their moods, and you are not seeing any beneficial changes, there's no shame in getting help from your senior counselor or their general physician. They may have answers for you regarding their mood changes, or see if it has to do with their medication or dosage. They may be able to recommend activities you try and get involved in, or therapies that have shown progress. It's okay to ask for help!

Chapter 12: Other Helpful Tips

Caring for someone who has dementia can be a struggle, and there is an initial learning process. Don't feel discouraged if you feel it's a tough job—because it is! This book is meant to provide you helpful suggestions and advice on how to handle certain situations, to reduce your stress and make it a more peaceful environment for you and your loved one with dementia.

Here are some other helpful tips that many caregivers have shared to help you on your journey.

Arguing may only make you both frustrated. It can be frustrating when your loved one is saying something untrue or repeating false stories or memories over and over. But you have to remind yourself it isn't them; it is dementia that is altering their mind. They truly believe what they are saying, because that is what their brain is telling them. You may be tempted to argue and correct them, but you cannot win an argument when someone's judgment and logic is altered. It may only end up in frustration for both of you and cause mood swings in your loved one. Remind yourself it's okay to let some battles go.

Cognitive activities are never a waste of time. It's never too late to try and improve your loved one's cognitive reasoning skills. It might seem sometimes like they're "too far gone," but remind yourself that at least you are spending time together, and you are making a memory with your loved one. Continue to work on things like puzzles, painting, arts and crafts, and whatever else it seems your loved one enjoys. These activities are always considered beneficial to dementia patients.

Prioritize what is most important to you and learn to relax about the rest. The simple matter is that patients with dementia are not going to be able to do everything perfectly. You have to learn what is most important to you as their caregiver. Maybe you prefer they take care of their physical hygiene. Or maybe it's more important to you that they are present at mealtimes with the family. Reassure your loved one and work with them constantly to help get through tasks that are most essential to you, and relax if things like exercise or creative activities have to be put on the back burner for a few days.

Sometimes space is all they need. If you notice a mood swing coming, or your loved one becoming combative or anxious, sometimes the best thing you can do is give them some space to calm down. First, be sure that they are safe if they go into their room, or any area they're in, but leave the room for 10 to 15 minutes so both of you can take a breath and re-examine the situation. You might find that when you come back to try a new approach, they are in a better mood and more willing to listen to what you say.

Stay educated on what medication your loved one is taking. Medications are often given to relieve symptoms of dementia, but your loved one may have other health conditions than dementia which requires medication, such as diabetes, high blood pressure, etc. One of the best things you can do is stay aware of their medication dosage, since more than likely, you are the one giving it to them. It's also important to have some basic understanding of how certain medications can affect the brain and possible side effects. This way, you will know if new behavior is related to medication or is something that should be brought to the doctor's attention. It's also essential that the doctor reviews any potential changes in your loved one's medication, supplements, dietary changes, and exercise routines. It's better to ask too many questions than not enough!

Have the tough conversations before you need. Topics like a will, living will, or power of attorney are daunting subjects to bring up with a loved one, because they only seem to remind us of our mortality. But talking about these choices and having the paperwork done before a medical emergency is crucial, so things aren't left unsettled. You want to be sure your loved one is still in the right frame of mind to answer these questions, and you feel satisfied enough by their answers. Most loved ones will feel a greater sense of peace to know their wishes will be honored.

Take care of yourself too! Caregiving can be a tough and exhausting job, especially if you're doing it alone or along with other responsibilities. Be sure you have a support system of people who can help when you are overwhelmed, and people you can talk to about the challenges you're facing. Along with other family members or friends, try to find a caregiver support group or a senior group at your local community center or retirement home. Give yourself breaks throughout the day, even if it's just an hour to yourself to unwind and relax when your loved one is taking a nap. Your health is very important too!

Conclusion

Thank for making it through to the end of *Alzheimer's and Dementia*. We hope this book was informative for you and able to provide you with many tips and tools as you diligently work as a caregiver to your loved one with dementia. Dementia can be a tasking disease that leaves everyone feeling exhausted and emotional. The best way to live with it is to have a routine and a safe environment where your loved one can be so you are not worried about their wellbeing. With our handy tips on making your home a safe place, you can ensure that you are creating the best environment for your loved one to feel comfortable, safe, and cared for.

The cognitive decline and emotions that come with dementia can be challenging, and it can be tough to communicate with someone who is having such difficulty relaying their feelings. We encourage you to be as positive as you can so your loved one can continue to feel calm and open towards you. Often, reacting with anger can make a situation worse. With help on how to safeguard your home, deal with wandering issues, create a healthy and balanced diet, and the importance of physical and mental exercise, you can begin to create a schedule that will help you and your loved one live a life of routine and less stress.

It's important to note that your health as the caregiver is very important. Be sure you have people to talk to, whether it's other family members, close friends, or a support group where you can talk about your frustrations and sadness. Your mental and physical health is very important, so be sure you are taking care of yourself and making your health a priority too.

Finally, if you found this book useful in any way, a review is always appreciated!

Jimmy D. Forest

Connect with us on our Facebook page www.facebook.com/bluesourceandfriends and stay tuned to our latest book promotions and free giveaways.

CPSIA information can be obtained
at www.ICGtesting.com
Printed in the USA
LVHW091936201220
674690LV00008B/1501